MW01291372

HEALTHY, HAPPY, WHOLE

Thirty days to a more balanced life

Alexandra MacKillop

www.AlexandraMacKillop.com

First Printing, 2019

EVERYTHING IN MODERATION

...even moderation.

Life is like a table. If you knock out one of the legs, the whole thing will crash to the ground. This is true no matter how beautifully it was decorated, how expensive it was, how many *good things* were placed upon it, or how well-constructed the other three legs were. For most of us, the tables of our lives are a little wobbly: family life is demanding, work is busy, and we're involved in numerous other activities that also consume our energy, time, and money. Nutrition and fitness (or other priorities) may fall by the wayside, and an unfriendly diagnosis might then compel us to look for a quick-fix weight-loss option. So, we metaphorically wrap some tape around the fracture in the table leg by going on a low-carb diet, hoping to lose some weight without having to think much about it. Maybe it will work, and maybe it won't, but regardless of the external outcome, it doesn't get to the root of the problem. It doesn't fix the broken table leg.

Dieting, fitness clubs and ministry retreats are just band-aids. They may boost morale for a short time, but they are nothing like the long-term, protective habits of intentional self-care in all areas of our lives. In cultivating new, healthful habits, baby steps prove themselves to be the most effective – time and time again. This book does not offer a total lifestyle transformation. It is not a quick fix, a guaranteed success to your greatest dreams, or a New

Year's Resolution. Instead, it offers details. It's the little things you can do within the existing template of your own life, while remaining cognizant of your own unique needs and values.

Savor it. Chew on it. Sit with it.

Take the time to consider the fine print of your own behaviors, attitudes, and beliefs and how they are affecting your ability to cultivate a happy, healthy, and holistically balanced life.

◆ ◆ ◆

How to Use This Resource

Healthy, Happy, Whole is a reflection guide that explores the integration of physical, mental/emotional, and spiritual health as applied to modern life. Each chapter is designed to be read on each of thirty days, consisting of a topic related to physical wellness, psychological well-being, and a devotional discussion of a chapter from the book of Proverbs. Each section culminates with a series of questions for self-reflection or group discussion. This guided study is a helpful tool for personal growth but is also well-suited for use in group bible studies, book studies, and mentorship meetings. It also can be used as an adjunct to other faith-forward wellness programs.

Why It Matters

The goal of this book is to help you cultivate awareness of the many complexities of well-being, which involve far more than a strict diet or rigid exercise schedule. If, in reading this book, you come to realize that your own habits are negatively affecting your life, please know that you're not alone. God sees you and hears you, and wants to offer you grace, hope, and life abundant. It may take time and practice to get there, but He is faithful!

Note: *If you are struggling to find balance with your own health, visit AlexandraMacKillop.com where you can learn more about cultivating the margin you need for a full, free, and faithful life.*

DAY 1

Healthy: Reframe Your Mindset
About Well-Being

When you think about health, what comes to mind? Do you visualize images of treadmills, green juice, and a life without donuts? Do you picture marathon training plans, nutrition labels, and long lists of what you should and shouldn't do? More often than not, rigid eating and exercise schedules aren't very effective in cultivating a healthier, more balanced life. In fact, anything that requires a sudden and extreme lifestyle upset often ends up being unsustainable. To make changes toward a healthier and more balanced life, small steps are far more effective for creating lasting results. In other words, less is more.

The word "health" is often associated with sterile, cold medical offices or viewed in association with some of the rigid regimes mentioned previously. Instead of striving toward "health," try reframing your mindset toward fostering your sense of *well-being*. This term is gentler and more holistic, encompassing the areas of life that are often neglected by diet and fitness schedules – things like emotional, relational, and spiritual wellness. Forming new habits is a slow process that requires patience and persistence, but when the goal is *well-being*, the results are always worth the effort. Well-being means cultivating lives that are less stressful, laying the foundation we need to truly become healthier people. It means spending time in activities that nourish our souls, changing the way we view wellness, and choosing to live in a way that honors our bodies for everything they were created to be.

1 When you've set out to make healthy changes in your life previously, were you successful? Why do you think you saw the results you did?

2 When you picture a life characterized by *well-being*, what comes to mind?

Happy: Foster Curiosity

Children have a way of viewing the world around them with awe and wonder. As adults, we often become jaded to the mysteries and intrigue of nature, science, faith, and friendship. We tend to become distracted by the hustle and bustle of life, bogged down by "the way things are" instead of pausing to consider *why things are that way*. As you begin to change your mindset towards health and well-being, it will become necessary to experiment with new ideas, consider new ways of thinking, and cultivate new practices that may feel challenging or stretching. By leaning into your sense of curiosity, you will be able to take steps towards the open-mindedness that is required for making change. When we are set in our ways, we become stagnant; when we start seeing new horizons, we are then able to reach them.

1 What excites you? What piques your interest? What would it mean to apply that same sense of curiosity towards the things that bore you?

2 What are some of your beliefs about health, wellness, happiness, and well-being that you've held for a long time? Which of these are you willing to consider changing?

Whole: Read Proverbs Chapter 1

Proverbs 1:7 reads: "The fear of the Lord is the beginning of knowledge, but fools despise wisdom and instruction." As much as we each might like to think otherwise, we don't know everything – we *can't*. There is always more to learn, more wisdom to acquire, more experience to gain. We each can grow, in one way or another, even if just to deepen our sense of understanding and empathy with others. Those with the most wisdom recognize the breadth of what they still have yet to learn. The one exception to this is God himself, who is the very beginning of wisdom. In this first chapter of Proverbs, we read about wisdom's many qualities, purposes, and applications. We see illustrations of those who lack wisdom, and are implored to be like those who seek to grow in wisdom by pursuing God.

1 Do you find that it is easy or difficult to admit when you don't know something, or if you have been wrong?

2 Have others pointed out areas you might benefit from changing your ways? How do you respond to instruction in these areas? What would it look like to respond differently?

DAY 2

Healthy: Go to the Doctor
When You're Not Sick

Most health insurance plans cover wellness checkups – annual medical physical exams for adults and children when they are healthy, fit, and well. Even though making an extra trip to the doctor's office might seem inconvenient, visiting with a physician when you *don't* have the flu can be extremely beneficial to your well-being. Here's why: Every person is unique, and baseline physical measures are different for every person. Ten different people can have different heights, weights, blood pressure measures, and cholesterol levels and still all be healthy.

However, if a person whose blood pressure usually falls into the low range of normal suddenly starts to have blood pressure at the high end of normal, this change is cause for concern. But if that person never knew what "normal" blood pressure means *for them as an individual,* emerging health problems could fly under the radar of their physicians until they become severe.

The purpose of preventative medicine is to identify risk factors and emerging health conditions before they become debilitating. However, when we neglect to visit the doctor for wellness check-ups, we miss out on the opportunity to have these baseline measurements and health screens performed. One of the best things we can do for our *future* well-being is make the choice to visit the doctor *today.*

1 Consider the health concerns that are currently affecting you or your family members. How would your or your family's health be better if those conditions had been identified sooner?

2 If annual physical exams at the doctor's office are not a part of your self-care routine, consider why that may be. What's stopping you from getting regular check-ups? What would inspire you to start?

Happy: De-Clutter

Alicia never thought of herself as a particularly disorganized person. She kept up with cleaning, washed her laundry on time, and she never was behind at work. But when she and her husband decided to move to another state, she was overwhelmed by the packing process. Somehow they had kept boxes of baby toys in their basement, and she *still* owned maternity pants even though her twin sons were already in high school. Her kitchen cabinets were stuffed with old Tupperware containers whose lids had been missing for years, and her drawers were ridden with socks that had been matchless for as long as she could remember. Somehow, the "little things" had piled up over time, and by the time the house was empty she and her husband had filled a dumpster with nearly as many items as their moving truck.

Clutter has a way of creating chaos. We don't always realize how the tension is building at the time, but suddenly it makes itself known: a stressful day that culminates with a shoe lost in an overflowing bin of footwear; the frantic search for a hair clip in a tangled box of hair accessories; the struggle to find something to wear in a packed closet of old, too small, or too-used clothes. It's amazing how liberating the process of de-cluttering and minimalizing can be. When we are able to pare down the items we don't want or need, we are set free to enjoy the simplicity of only owning what truly brings us joy.

1 Which items do you find it difficult to get rid of – even if they don't serve a function in your life? Why do you think that is?

2 What area of your life can you commit to de-cluttering *today*?

Whole: Read Proverbs Chapter 2

The first chapter of Proverbs explains the utility of wisdom, and this second chapter strengthens the case for cultivating a life that is rooted in knowledge of the ways of God. We read that if we "call out for insight" and "cry out for understanding," if we search diligently for it, "as for silver" or hidden treasure, then we will grow in wisdom.

The process of gaining knowledge from God is two-fold. On one hand, we must desire it. We need to understand the importance of wise living so that we can whet our appetites for it. On the other hand, we must take action. Growing in the wisdom of God can take many forms, many of which involve learning directly from others. Examples may include attending church, consulting with different mentors in our lives or those we look up to, or dedicated study of God's word. Gaining wisdom takes work, but the reward for our efforts is enormous.

1 What practices in your daily life enable you to grow in wisdom? If you don't have any currently, what would it look like to implement some?

2 Who are some individuals with whom a friendship would allow you to gain wisdom? Which relationships can you deepen for the purpose of growing in godly insight?

DAY 3

Healthy: Rate Your Hunger

Most folks start new diets because they're looking for a simple solution: *"If I avoid this one thing,"* they think, *"Then I can eat as much as I want of everything else."* But the problem faced by most people who struggle with their weight isn't that they're eating the "wrong things." More often than not, they are eating too much – and the reason is because they aren't "tuned in" to their hunger signals.

When we mindlessly eat – distracted, stressed, or multitasking – we aren't able to identify when our hunger dissipates. We eat and eat until the portion is gone, regardless of whether we've reached the point of satisfaction. When we aren't satisfied, stopping eating feels harder. But when we are aware of our hunger signals, present with our food, and listening for the body cues that tell us we are full, it's easier to stop eating at the appropriate time. With mindful eating, we can walk away from a meal both full *and* satisfied.

Before you sit down to a meal, rate your hunger on a scale of 0 to 10, where 0 signifies a famished feeling, and 10 is *Thanksgiving stuffed*. Continue eating until you're satisfied, and again, identify where on the 0-10 scale your fullness falls. Reflect on how much food you needed to move forward on the scale as you did. Repeat this exercise every time you eat, or as often as you remember. The more often you do it, the more beneficial it will be.

Happy: Schedule a Sabbath

In the times of the Old Testament, refraining from work, school, and other typical responsibilities on weekly Sabbath days was *forbidden*. This law was part of an agreement between God and his people to establish holiness and remind the Israelites of the difference between *their sinfulness* and *His perfection*. Thanks to the sacrifice of Jesus on the cross, we are no longer bound to the laws of the Old Testament. However, in many ways, observing those principles can still serve to benefit us, today. For example, the cleanliness rituals of handwashing and dish washing were helpful for the Israelites whose limited understanding of micro-biology might have otherwise strengthened the spread of disease.

The concept of a Sabbath rest can be viewed likewise in today's busy modern age. In our culture, we are overscheduled, overridden with responsibilities, and often exhausted. Setting aside the workweek responsibilities every Sunday to rest in God can be of enormous benefit to us in all areas of our lives.

1 How do you typically spend your Sundays? Do you find that these habits help you to de-stress, or do they contribute to your stress? Do they strengthen your relationship with God, or do they create distance?

2 If a whole day of Sabbath rest sounds overwhelming, start small: What is one thing you typically do on Sundays that you can commit to resting from for the foreseeable future?

Whole: Read Proverbs Chapter 3

Proverbs 3:6 reads: "In all your ways, submit to him, and he will make straight your paths." Imagine you've decided to run a marathon. So, you visit your local library and check out every DVD about marathons, training, and running that you can find. Then, you plop down on the couch and start watching.Sitting on the couch is not a very effective means for growing in the endurance and athleticism required to run a marathon. In fact, it creates a huge barrier to successful running!

We often tend to do the same thing in our faith. We find that our ways seem crooked, and so we become frustrated with God because he isn't doing what we expect him to do in a given situation. We may feel we are doing the right thing – living His way – but unknowingly, our approach in another area is a little off. Just like watching DVD's about running is *related* to the subject at hand but ineffective for training, some areas of our lives that are unrelated to the area of prayer may be evading our awareness. Failing to honor God in just one area of life can affect all other areas.

1   What are the areas of your life that you struggle to submit to God? For example, do you have an iron grip around money and subsequently neglect to tithe?

2   Are you holding a grudge against someone from your past? Is there someone from whom you need to ask forgiveness?

3   If we think we've surrendered our lives to God and things aren't working out as we expect, it could be that we never fully surrendered at all.

DAY 4

Healthy: Decide to Ditch Dieting

Have you ever sought out a "quick fix" to one of your problems? With dieting, this is exactly what we are hoping to accomplish. Diets promise weight loss as an easy consequence of following a strict set of eating rules. But the problem is that diets can't fulfill their promises. They fail almost every time. Albert Einstein is credited with describing insanity as doing the same thing over and over again but expecting different results. If you've tried diet after diet in attempt to control your weight and have been failed by your efforts time and time again, the next right response probably isn't another diet.

Giving up on a lifestyle of dieting means giving up on the search for a "quick fix" for weight loss. It means putting in the time and effort to reconcile with our bodies' hunger and fullness cues, learning how to respond appropriately to our internal signals, respecting the role of food in our lives, honoring our bodies, and submitting to the fact that real results require hard work and time. By cultivating attunement to our bodies, we can maintain good health without falling into a harmful yo-yo diet cycle again and again.

1 Think about the last time you went on a diet. How did it end? Did it ultimately make your life better and help you accomplish your goals? Is your life better *today* because of those previous efforts?

2 What is standing in the way of you and a diet-free life? Do you struggle with fears? Shame? Guilt? Be honest with yourself and take the time to understand what drives *you* individually toward seeking out "quick fixes" in your health.

Happy: Question What You Consume

Often, our behaviors stem from our beliefs, and our beliefs stem from what we allow to influence us. The more we allow ourselves to be exposed to worldviews that clash with our own, the more likely we are to yield to outside pressures that are contrary to our own values. An excellent way to protect your heart from ideas and exposures that could lead you down a road you don't desire is by embarking on a social media cleanse. It looks like this:

Write out a mission statement for your life. Perhaps you are passionate about leading others to Christ, sharing knowledge, cultivating beauty, or minimizing your carbon foot print. Then, sift through everyone you follow on social media and unfollow accounts that share messages that don't align with your mission statement.

1 How do you feel after reading negative messages, public complaints, or ideas that conflict with your values?

2 Protect yourself from these joy-draining influences by filtering your social media. Who will you unfollow?

Whole : Read Proverbs Chapter 4

Have you ever noticed that after hanging around a certain friend or family member, you start to act like that person?

17

Whether good or bad, the influences we allow into our lives eventually come to shape who we are. Proverbs 4:23 reads: "Above all else, guard your heart, for everything you do flows from it." What this means is that our words, thoughts, and actions are an outflowing of our hearts. What we come to know and love effectively translates into our behaviors and attitudes. When we aren't careful to guard against harmful influences in our lives, they can sneak in and start wreaking havoc on us, spiritually.

1 Which activities tend to prompt you to behave, think, or respond differently than God would have you behave, think, or respond to others?

2 How can you set boundaries in those areas to limit your exposure or influence, thereby protecting your heart, from which everything you do flows?

DAY 5

Healthy: Identify What
You Really Need

How often do we turn to distractions when we are wrestling with uncomfortable emotions, or to food when we are tired, cranky, or stressed? How often do we pick fights with our loved ones when the root cause of our frustration is loneliness, or buy more *stuff* as a means for *stuffing down* our worries? Nearly every problem in life could be avoided if instead of turning to unproductive coping mechanisms, we practiced honest identification of our needs and chose to respond in kind.

When you find yourself turning to unhealthy behaviors, commit to uncovering the underlying cause of that behavior. Which uncomfortable emotions prompt your desire to self-soothe in unproductive ways? Instead of resorting to shame and blame when things don't go as planned, take honest inventory of yourself and your actions, and commit to self-care instead of self-sabotage through unhealthy behavior.

1 Which bad behaviors do you find yourself struggling with time after time?

2 Think back on the last time or two you engaged in this behavior: what was your emotional state? Were you hungry, stressed, or grieving?

3 How could you have better responded to those needs?

Happy: Self-Reflection

In the same way that we can engage in honest self-reflection after our wayward decisions, we can help prevent such unfortunate situations by engaging in a daily process of self-reflection. By checking in with ourselves and allowing the space to reconcile with our mental, emotional, physical, and spiritual needs, we can prevent problems from getting out of hand. If we identify the early rumblings of boredom coming on, we can get up and get moving for a breath of fresh air or a change of scenery. Left unchecked, boredom could lead to boredom eating, loneliness, or a dark tunnel of social media or other time wasters.

1 What are you feeling right now, in this moment? Ask yourself this question throughout the day – perhaps in the morning and afternoon lulls when you start finding yourself tempted to engage in unhealthy behavior.

2 Consider keeping a journal by your bed and jot down the times in your day when you experienced highs and lows. Re-read these entries and see if you can identify any patterns. What can you do to change those patterns in the moments that they emerge?

Whole: Read Proverbs Chapter 5

Proverbs 5:21 reads: "For your ways are in full view of the Lord, and he examines all your paths." God is omniscient. This means that he is constantly aware of the happenings of the world, the happenings in our minds, and the happenings in our hearts. Although we may struggle on an individual level to understand our behaviors and feelings, God is already aware of them. He knows what we will feel before we feel it, and he knows why. He knows what we will do before we do it, and he knows when.

The fact that we are known deeply and intimately by the God who created us is an enormously freeing truth. When we struggle to understand ourselves, we can turn to the one who already does, and ask him for wisdom, guidance, and strength to take the next right step. Another facet of God's omniscience is that he can't be fooled. Even when we trick ourselves into thinking we are eating a snack out of hunger when it's really out of boredom, God can't be led to believe falsehoods. We can't trick him into believing the same lies that we use to excuse ourselves of our behavior. The more you spend time in God's word, the better you will be able to identify right and wrong, and the less likely you will be to try to trick yourself into living outside of God's will – your ways are always in His full view.

1 Do you find it difficult to identify what's going on in your head and your heart when you make choices you aren't proud of? Ask God to help you gain clarity.

2 What are some of the lies you tell yourself in an attempt to excuse your behavior?

DAY 6

Healthy: Drink More Water

The human body is 60% water – scientists estimate that the brain and heart are nearly 75% water, the lungs weigh in at 83%, and even skin is 64% water. Every breath we take expels water vapor, and with more than 23,000 breaths taken per day, we are losing incredible amounts of fluid just through restful activities. Current recommendations for hydration encourage a fluid intake that is much higher than most of us are getting – one ounce for every kilogram of body weight. To calculate how much water you should be drinking daily, divide your body weight (in pounds) by two, and then divide that number by 8. This gives you the number of eight-ounce glasses of water you should expect to replenish each day.

If you struggle to reach that level of water intake, consider carrying a water bottle with you throughout your day. Switch to decaf coffee, choose herbal tea, or seltzer to add flavor if you find yourself getting bored. Water empowers our very lives, so getting enough each day is crucial for our well-being.

1 How much water should *you* be drinking each day? Are you getting that much? If not, what can you do *today* to improve your hydration?

2 Consider downloading a health-tracking app to monitor your water intake for a few days and see where you need to grow.

Happy: Just Do It

The athletic brand *Nike* is famous for it's motivating slogan: "Just do it." The three words speak to the fact that regardless of how uncomfortable something is and regardless of how tempting procrastination seems, if something needs to be done, the best course of action is to just buckle down and get it done. Sometimes we accumulate long lists of responsibilities, and the more we push them away, the more they accumulate. As with clutter, little by little, our to-do lists grow until one day we become completely overwhelmed by them.

The stress and exhaustion of such high demand can drive some people to their breaking points. One of the best ways to keep to-do lists manageable is to avoid procrastination. When the need becomes known, take care of it right away. Instead of flagging emails, respond to them immediately, then archive them. If a doctor's appointment needs to be scheduled, do it right away. By *doing the thing right now*, we increase our level of productivity and are able to minimize the psycho-emotional fallout that results from procrastination.

1 Which items on your to-do list have been there the longest? What has gotten in the way of you accomplishing them? Make a plan *today* to conquer that task.

2 Some to-do list items are left unfinished because they aren't also high on our priority lists. Sometimes tasks are low on the priority list because they aren't actually that important. Clutter on our to-do lists can be as damaging to our mental health as procrastination. If it isn't something that actually needs to be part of your life, toss it out and move on with the more important things.

Whole: Read Proverbs Chapter 6

Don't put off to tomorrow what needs to be done today. Part of stewarding our lives well means taking initiative in planning for the future, providing for today, and learning from the past. Neglecting our responsibilities, putting off necessary changes, and ignoring the big red flags can lay way for sudden disaster. Without savings, a car wreck could wreck you financially, too. Without a solid baseline of health, catching the flu could wipe you off your feet for twice as long as a person for whom wellness is a priority. Without addressing the nagging arguments in your marriage, a sudden, unforseen stressor could tear your relationship completely apart.

In this chapter of Proverbs, verses 10 and 11 urge us not to neglect our responsibilities for the allure of a little more leisure. While rest certainly is a necessary part of life, failing to take initiative will harm us, too. Everything seems fine until it isn't anymore.

1 Is there something you've been neglecting to do, which may cause problems if left unchecked for too long? What can you do *today* to start making progress in this area?

2 Who can you consult for objective advice and wisdom about your priorities in life? Humbly ask a trusted friend or mentor to speak into your life and priorities, helping you cultivate awareness about areas you can grow.

DAY 7

Healthy: Vitamin D

When's the last time you had your vitamin D levels checked? For most folks, the answer is probably *never*. But what most folks also don't realize is that vitamin D deficiency, in addition to being extremely widespread, is extremely dangerous. Deficiencies of vitamin D are associated with depression, cancer, cardiovascular disease, osteoporosis, cognitive decline, hormonal imbalances, asthma, diabetes, and more!

Unlike most vitamins, which we can receive in adequate levels from food, our natural sources of vitamin D don't come from food – they come from the sun! But with indoor nine-to-five jobs, schooling, long winters, and knowledge of harmful UV rays, our exposure to the sun is limited. So, in order to receive the dosage needed for health and well-being, most adults need to supplement this nutrient. However, vitamin D supplementation also comes with a risk of overdose.

Unlike certain vitamins and minerals with which excess can be safely eliminated from the body, excesses of vitamins A, D, E and K are stored in body fat. Too little vitamin D is dangerous, but so is too *much* vitamin D. Supplementing with a daily multivitamin is recommended for most folks, but even this amount often isn't sufficient to prevent deficiency. The best way to promote healthy vitamin D levels is to have your levels checked, and for a primary healthcare provider to oversee your supplement protocol. A licensed physician can help you return to a healthy vitamin

D level safely.

1 Vitamin deficiencies may seem like a problem of the past, but they're far more common in today's society than many folks realize. Don't let your health suffer because you neglected to check your vitamin D levels.

2 Make an appointment for a "fit and well" exam at your primary healthcare provider's office today and ask for a blood test.

Happy: 5 Minute Meditation

If you write 150 words each day (three sentences), by the end of a year you will have written an entire book. If you walk one mile every day, you'll have finished a marathon in less than a month. If you save $3 every day (say, a coffee at Dunkin Donuts), by the end of a year you will have saved more than $1,000. It's shocking how powerful something *small* can be.

Learning to meditate seems like an impossible feat. But throughout scripture and history, we read of the benefits and importance of meditation. In Psalm 199 verse 97, we read: "Oh, how I love your law! I meditate on it all day long." But there's no need to meditate for an entire day. Just start with 5 minutes. Go to a quiet place, close your eyes, and pray. Concentrate on God's goodness, on his commands, on his provision in your life. You will be amazed by what 5 minutes can do.

When will you fit in a five-minute meditation *today*?

Whole : Read Proverbs Chapter 7

Have you ever found yourself humming along to an old tune that was popular *years* ago? The mind is an amazing creation in terms of its incredible ability to learn and remember information. These memories sometimes pop up when we least expect them, just like hearing just a short segment of a song on the radio can leave us singing the whole lyric.

Meditating on scripture and committing verses to memory is an excellent way to equip our hearts with positive and encouraging truths, which the holy spirit will bring to mind at unexpected times. It's amazing how God uses the return on such investments for our good and His glory. If scripture memory isn't a regular part of your life, commit to changing that!

1 Have you ever memorized scripture? Do you still know those verses by heart today? Reflect on how amazing it is that God can bring those words to your attention with such little prompting.

2 Start today by memorizing Proverbs 7:1.

DAY 8

Healthy: Cook at Home

Fast food is fun sometimes, but most folks would agree that it isn't necessarily a good thing to eat every day. In addition to crowding out the nutritious foods we need to be eating on a daily basis, frequenting fast food locations can also have a negative impact on our wallets. Cooking at home is a great way to include healthy foods in our diets on a regular basis. It also is less expensive than buying prepared meals, and can be a fun pastime as a date night or as a way to engage the family in a collaborative project.

Cooking is creative, healthful, and can foster close relationships when done together. Plus, leftovers are the homecooked equivalent to fast food, but unlike McDonald's is much more nutritious. There's no good reason *not* to cook at home regularly. If you need recipe inspiration, check out a cookbook from the library, peruse new ideas on Pinterest, or ask friends and family for their favorites.

1 Are most of your meals eaten on the go or at home? Do you typically buy pre-made meals or do you cook from scratch? Why do you think that is?

2 Commit to cooking one new recipe this week. When will you buy the ingredients? Which day will you cook? Who will you invite? Plan the details *now* so that you can make sure it happens *later*.

Happy: Prioritize Family

As with all relationships, family relationships require an enormous investment of time, energy, and effort. But *unlike* other relationships, the bond among siblings, parents, grandparents, and children is deeper than just a choice. Our families don't define who we are, but through their love and support, they can empower us to be the best versions of who we are. For most of us, our families are always around us, and it can be easy to take them for granted. But those who are closest to us are the ones we should treat with the most care and intention, investing in them the most.

When God calls us to love others as ourselves, the first and closest people he tasks us with are our families: parents, siblings, spouses, and children. Loving our families well makes them stronger and better able to pour out that love into the community, whereas families that are struggling to be unified cannot serve as far and as wide or have as great of an impact as that which comes from a unified group. Husbands, love and serve your wives. Wives, love and serve your husbands. Parents, invest in your children, teaching them the ways that should go. Children, honor and obey your parents. Christians, love, serve, honor, and invest in your families, strengthening them to go and do likewise.

1 Which conflicts do you tend to see over and over again in your home? Have a family meeting to assess the health of your relationships. As always, approach this with a humble spirit, inviting feedback and being honest about your feelings.

2 What can you do today to foster closeness and friendship with your spouse, parents, children, or grandparents? Invest in a strong relationship now; the benefits will pay off later.

Whole: Read Proverbs Chapter 8

What do you desire most in life? Love? Money? Confidence? Happiness? The bible isn't an instruction manual, and it certainly doesn't promise that following God will grant us our every whim and desire. But it *does* teach us that cultivating a life centered on the things of God – his wisdom, knowledge, and love – will shape us to desire the things he desires, love the things he loves, and live as he designed for us to live. In order to do these things, we need to seek wisdom.

While wise living won't necessarily find us a new job or help us win the lottery, it will teach us how to cultivate meaningful relationships and steward our money well. While wisdom won't change our beauty or social status, it will give us the confidence we need to go forward in life boldly for Christ, and to find joy in a life lived well. In Proverbs 8:11 we read: "For wisdom is more precious than rubies, and nothing you desire can compare with her." The allure of worldly values is incomparable to the gift and gratification of wise living under God.

1 How are you currently seeking to grow in Christ? How do you assess whether your actions are consistent with God's calling on your life to live wisely?

2 The best place to find wisdom is the bible. How often do you spend time reading God's word? What would it look like to strengthen this pattern in your life?

DAY 9

Healthy: When You Eat, Eat

Are you a multitasker? Most people are, at least when they're eating. But the distractions of scrolling through a phone, watching TV, reading the paper, working, or driving when eating can make it difficult to stay attuned to the process of nourishing ourselves. When we're not paying attention, we can't listen very well – so when we aren't paying attention *to our bodies* when we are eating, we can't *perceive hunger and fullness signals* very well.

Have you ever been so hungry that you ate your food too quickly to even taste it? Distracted eating can cause the same phenomenon. If we aren't perceiving that we're eating throughout the process of a meal, it's likely that we will finish eating and feel full but not *satisfied*. When you eat, do your best to avoid distractions. Leave the work at your desk, turn off the TV, put away your phone. Focus on your food so that you can taste every mouthful. Engage with your meals and allow them to fully nourish you rather than simply fill your belly.

1 Which times of day do you find yourself most tempted to disengage during meals?

2 What will you do *today* to minimize distractions while you are eating?

Happy: Learn to Savor

Do you feel guilty for eating a brownie? How about for watching TV? What about for spending a few extra dollars out on a date night? Where is this guilt coming from? Because it's not from God. There's nothing immoral about enjoying dessert or a choice pastime. There's nothing wrong with choosing to spend your money on special experiences with your loved ones. Sure, we all *could* stand to eat another salad, turn off the TV, or save a little extra cash. But life is meant to be lived, and all these experiences are little blessings that bring us joy.

While there's certainly *more to life* than pleasure, there's also no need to shame ourselves for pleasant experiences. Most of the things we guilt ourselves for are completely benign subjects. We create rules about them for ourselves, and there's absolutely nobody higher that is holding us accountable in the same way. What if we chose to live with fewer rules, embraced the freedom of God, and decided to ditch guilt, once and for all?

1 What are the things you most often find yourself feeling guilty for enjoying? Where do you think this guilt comes from?

2 If the behaviors that leave you ashamed compromise your values, what would it look like to take steps towards turning from the immoral behavior once and for all?

3 Who could you ask for accountability or advice in this area so that you can be set free from the guilt and heal your heart?

Whole: Read Proverbs Chapter 9

Let's rewind a few days to Proverbs 4:7, which reads: "The beginning of wisdom is this: get wisdom." This verse points to the truth that in order for someone to be able to grow in wisdom, they need to have some sort of interest in becoming wiser. Without that fundamental desire, it's impossible for them to have the motivation to learn. We see a similar paradigm in Proverbs 9:8 – "Do not rebuke mockers or they will hate you; rebuke the wise and they will love you."

If a person has no desire to change their ways, pointing out an area for them to improve is futile; they will likely reject your advice. In the same vein, individuals who are constantly seeking to improve themselves welcome opportunities to reflect, hear constructive criticism, and reform their ways. An important facet of wisely sharing knowledge is knowing when it is and isn't appropriate.

1 How do you typically respond when others offer you correction? Do you respond with hostility and defensiveness, or with a humble, coachable spirit?

2 If you are not as receptive to feedback as you might like to be, ask God to help you understand why you respond as you do so that you can answer more gracefully in the future.

DAY 10

Healthy: Be Prepared

What do you think poses more of a health risk: eating too much or eating too little? Though it may be surprising – considering the advertising we're exposed to in today's day and age – being under-fed is actually more harmful to health than having too much food. While the most commonly known risk of eating too little is malnourishment in the form of vitamin deficiencies, long-term calorie deficits can lead to multisystem organ failure, neurologic damage, and even death. In the short term, inadequate nutrition can create a predisposition to developing diabetes, cardiovascular disease, and other conditions.

One of the major contributing factors to these diseases is from poor blood sugar control, which results when a person's carbohydrate intake is not adequately balanced by consumption of protein, fiber, and nutritious snacks. Long stretches between meals, especially without enough protein, can cause blood sugar to drop and then spike at the next meal. These patterns can lead to insulin resistance and also create inflammation, which is an enormous contributor to cardiovascular disease. Of course, eating fast food during these "hunger emergencies" isn't always the best choice either. So, the best way to combat them is to carry high protein snacks in purses, backpacks, cars, and briefcases. In this case, an ounce of prevention is literally worth a pound of cure!

1 Do you find yourself getting too hungry between meals? What does hunger (or low blood sugar) feel like to you? Pay attention to your body so you can recognize these signals sooner.

2 Where in your life can you stash high-protein snacks for easy access? Will they be easy to find during the times you are most likely to need them?

Happy: Reverse the Equation

When we feel happy, we generally smile. When we feel down in the dumps, we generally frown. Smiling when we're feeling badly just doesn't seem to make sense. Or does it? On days when everything seems to be going wrong, painting on a happy face doesn't come easily, and it certainly isn't our natural instinct. But what's amazing is that intentionally changing the expressions on our faces can reverse the equation and actually help stimulate our brains to activate the neurological pathways associated with positive emotions. In other words, instead of happiness leading to smiling, smiling can help lead to happiness! Or, at the very least, it can perk up someone's mood and serve as a blessing to those passing by. (Seeing a smiling face on the sidewalk or at the store is always a more pleasant sight than looking upon a downcast soul.)

1 Which types of things typically make you feel stressed out or down in the dumps? Write a note to yourself as a reminder to smile when you're not feeling like it. Leave it in a place you know you'll see it.

2 Sometimes our natural instincts aren't always what's best for us. What are some of your other emotional or behavioral "default modes" that you might consider actively reversing?

Whole: Read Proverbs Chapter 10

If you have children or younger siblings, you know from experience that they are watching you. Young children pick up the patterns of those around them, modeling the behavior they see and repeating the words they hear. Therefore, we generally try to be on our best behavior around children so that they model and repeat *positive* behaviors and speech.

As Christians – whether we are young or old – the world is watching us. They are waiting to see our every move, wondering how we will respond to everything from global events to personal conversation. For those who are new to the faith, observing mature Christians putting faith into practice can be an enormous encouragement if done well, or a huge impediment to personal growth if done poorly. Proverbs 10:17 reads, "Whoever heeds discipline shows the way to life, but whoever ignores correction leads others astray." When we live rightly, we are able to inspire others to do likewise. But when we fall into our own patterns of sin, let our guard down against the ways of the world, we set a terrible example for others, who are watching us.

1 When you were a new Christian, were there individuals you looked up to, whose faith inspired you? Which qualities were encouraging?

2 How would your behavior or word choices be different if you were constantly aware that others were watching? How would they be different if you were constantly aware that *God* is watching?

3 How can you seek to model your faith to those around you?

DAY 11

Healthy: Cut Back on Caffeine

In addition to under eating or skipping meals, caffeine is another contributing factor to blood sugar swings. The reason that coffee and tea help us feel energized is because caffeine activates our "fight or flight" system. While it's helpful for getting up and getting going, activating this nervous response creates chemical stress. Over time, this elevated stress level can harm our health. It also can harm our health by masking over other symptoms that might be important indicators of bad habits. For example, not getting enough sleep has been linked to poor memory, disease risk, and other health problems.

Masking over tiredness with coffee can create the false illusion of well-being when we really aren't well at all. Consuming too much caffeine can also be problematic because it is a diuretic, which means it dehydrates us. Remember the discussion about hydration? Each cup of coffee counts *against* a person's daily water goal. While moderate consumption of caffeinated beverages can be part of a healthy lifestyle, too much of them can create health risks.

1 Consider your consumption of caffeinated beverages. Why are you drinking them? Is it to make up for a sleep deficit? To serve as a meal replacement? For an afternoon energy boost during episodes of nutrition-related fatigue?

2 If you find that your use of caffeine is excessive or improper, consider cutting back your consumption.

Current FDA recommendation is to not exceed 400 mg of caffeine per day.

Happy: Donate Time

At the end of our lives, the most important investments we will have made will be those involving the people in our lives. That's right – not the money we earned, the stuff we owned, or any of our accomplishments. The greatest treasures here on earth are those which will follow us to heaven: our relationships. Donating money to charity is a wonderful thing to do, and millions of lives are positively impacted each day from such donations. But even more impactful than giving ten dollars is the gift of love.

Donating time to serve others not only creates the opportunity to meet practical needs but can also be a doorway into sharing encouragement through faith. Visiting at a retirement home, serving at a soup kitchen, volunteering at church, or joining a buddy program for individuals with special needs are all extremely important but often overlooked tasks – many of which require a greater sacrifice than writing a check, but offer a far more extensive reward.

1 Reflect on a time when someone has invested personally in your life. How have you benefitted from that person's sacrifice of time and other resources? What would it look like to pay that investment forward?

2 Which organizations in your area are in need of volunteer time to run? How can you become involved in these organizations on a weekly or monthly basis?

Whole: Read Proverbs Chapter 11

"A kindhearted woman gains honor, but ruthless men gain only wealth." – Proverbs 11:16

Who would you rather be friends with: someone who is well-respected, kind, and selfless, or someone who uses others for personal gain? Hopefully the answer to this question is obvious. Nobody wants to spend time with people who are selfish, hurtful, and inconsiderate, and most of us would be grieved to learn that others thought that way of us. But on the other hand, are we intentional about expressing kindness, encouraging others, and serving our communities? Reading the bible, we can easily fall into a place of self-righteousness, thanking God that we aren't the terrible "ruthless" individuals He warns against – or are we?

1 Consider your daily interactions with the people in your life. Would they describe you as kindhearted? Why or why not?

2 How does a kindhearted person behave? What types of words do they use? What is their attitude like? What would it look like for you to act and think likewise?

DAY 12

Healthy: Cultivate a Walking Practice

Exercise is an important piece of a healthy lifestyle, but it doesn't need to take the form of a gym membership to be beneficial. Simple tasks like playing with children, vigorously cleaning the home, and fast-paced shopping all offer the same physical benefits as other types of exercise. With physical activity, the biggest consideration is sustainability.

Walking is a wonderful form of exercise for a few reasons: First of all, it can be done pretty much anywhere. There is no equipment required (except maybe a good pair of shoes) and it can fit into even the busiest of schedules. Whether it's a leisurely half-hour stroll or a few quick laps around campus a couple times of day, it's the simple steps that add up to make a significant difference. Second, walking is excellent because there's no prep-work or clean-up required. A sweaty jog warrants a shower before getting back to work, but provided the season is right (or a treadmill is available) a person can literally walk right into the next task on their to-do list.

Taking a walk every day is an easy way to add physical activity to your day without a huge commitment of time, money, or mental energy. Aim for 30 minutes per day, and bring your dog, spouse, family, or a friend. It's an excellent way to invest in social relationships while getting an added health benefit at the same time!

1 When in your day do you have a spare 10-30 minutes to take a walk?

2 What do you need in order to be successful with a daily walking practice? New shoes? A new friend?

Happy: Team Building

Everywhere we look, strength is in the numbers. Herds of elephants can conquer lions; colonies of ants can carry loads fifty times their weight; thousands of cables together can suspend the golden gate bridge – none of these feats would be possible on an individual level, but through togetherness they can be accomplished.

Ecclesiastes 4:12 reads: "Though one may be overpowered, two can defend themselves. A cord of three strands is not quickly broken." With God in the picture, then the miraculous becomes possible.

1 What are some of your current goals for well-being? Which friend will you ask to join you? Read this book together. Commit to a walking route together. Hold each other accountable in cutting back on caffeine.

2 The third strand in the cord described by Ecclesiastes 4:12 is God. Are your goals – whether as applicable to well-being or otherwise – consistent with his calling on your life? Pray through them and ask Him for guidance in pointing you toward His glory.

Whole: Read Proverbs Chapter 12

When our friends and family members give us advice, we tend to trust them. Being in relationship with our loved ones for long periods of time gives us insight into their values, desires, and habits. We can trust our friends because we *know* them – we've seen who they are in real life, and if their patterns of behavior are encouraging to us, we likely try to emulate them. Taking advice from just anyone, however, isn't always the best idea. Even if they are well-meaning, individuals who don't share our worldview may encourage us in certain ways that ultimately lead down roads we would rather not be on, long term.

When seeking advice, be sure to consult individuals who not only share your faith but who also have exhibited Godly behavior consistently over time. These are the type of people who likely can be trusted to give advice that would point you toward the type of life you ultimately would desire to live under God. When we read Proverbs 12:5, we understand that there are two types of people: those who live according to God's will, and those who don't. This is why we must exercise caution in taking advice because sometimes, it isn't clear who belongs with whom. "The plans of the righteous are just, but the advice of the wicked is deceitful."

1 Where do you usually turn when you are seeking advice or wisdom in decision-making?

2 Who are the people in your life whose behavior, attitudes, and lifestyles you'd like to emulate? How can you cultivate a closer relationship with these individuals to encourage you in your faith?

DAY 13

Healthy: Add One More

Healthful eating doesn't need to be complicated. We simply need to eat enough food, in substantial quantities with an abundance of healthful vitamins and minerals. But in order to cultivate a practice of balanced eating, doing so needs to be desirable. Many folks avoid vegetables because they feel they aren't as satisfying as other choices, but that doesn't need to be the case. Prepared well, vegetables can become something you truly crave with regularity. Not only do they offer the micronutrients that are necessary for good health, but they add flavor, fiber, and more to meals.

Today, strive to add one more vegetable to your day. A handful of spinach in a smoothie, some tomatoes with scrambled eggs, extra carrots in soup – all of these are easy and virtually unnoticeable additions. But the best way to get more veggies is to learn to prepare them in a way that's enjoyable for what they are. Vegetables should taste good, and with this easy recipe, they can.

Recipe for Roasted Vegetables:
1) Choose a vegetable to prepare. Anything works – seriously, *anything.*
2) Pre-heat the oven to 300 degrees Fahrenheit.
3) Line a cookie sheet with foil.
4) Prepare 3 cups of vegetables: this is the equivalent of one bag of frozen, pre-sliced vegetables, or fresh vegetables cut

into ½-inch slices.

5) Toss the vegetables in olive oil, salt, and pepper – 1 table-spoon of oil per cup of vegetables, salt and pepper to taste. (Add garlic powder, chili flakes, or soy sauce for a flavor twist!)

6) If the vegetables were frozen or are root vegetables, cook for about 25 minutes, to desired tenderness. If the vegetables were fresh, cook for about 15-20 minutes.

7) Enjoy!

Which vegetable will you be adding today?

Happy: Reverse-Scheduling

Have you ever gotten home at the end of a long day, irritated and exhausted yet completely unsure of how you fell into such downheartedness? In most cases, little things pile up through-out the day, affecting our attitudes and our emotions, dragging us down little by little until we suddenly realize we are in a sour mood with little concept of how we arrived there. Often, this is the result of overscheduling, too many demands, and too little time to process through the little hiccups that cause strife. Awareness is the first step in making change. To better under-stand the demands that are bringing down your day, use this re-verse scheduling exercise:

Make a daily time chart that starts at the time you wake up and ends at the time you go to bed, divided into 30-minute inter-vals. Every day for one week, write down what you're doing at the beginning of every thirty-minute interval, and for how long you worked on that activity. This should include everything from showering to eating, from scrolling social media to work meet-ings. The more detail, the better. At the end of the week, add up how much time you spent doing each respective task. If your schedule is heavily weighted towards things that bring you down (such as screen time, time spent in an unhealthy work environment, etc.) it may be time to make some changes.

W hat is taking more time in your week than it deserves? How can you cut back on these life-draining activities and better allocate that time toward full and free living?

Whole: Read Proverbs Chapter 13

Do you ever take short cuts? Or rather, have you ever tried to take a short cut only to find out that it wasn't a short cut at all? Students may copy their friends' homework; but when exam time rolls around, it's clear that they never learned the information. A late driver may speed to work, only to get pulled over along the way, adding back all the time they tried to save *and then some*.

A dieter may start up a new program to lose weight quickly, but ultimately find their efforts to be unsustainable. They give up, gain back the weight, and six months later find themselves worse off than if they'd made small changes gradually over time. "Dishonest money dwindles away, but whoever gathers money little by little makes it grow," is what we read in Proverbs 13:11. The right course of action may not appear to be the easiest, fastest, or most effective. *In the beginning.* But as time passes, the slow and steady, righteous way is always the best. As Christians in today's day and age, we may not be robbers, swindlers, or dishonest salesmen. But are we looking for other shortcuts?

1 Where in your life have you taken shortcuts that turned out to be longer, riskier, or otherwise more challenging than the righteous way?

2 Which types of situations cause you to feel the temptation to take a shortcut? Which types of emotions do you feel in those circumstances? Are there certain patterns of behavior or choices that tend to lead up to those desperate moments?

DAY 14

Healthy: Learn to Savor

As a child, did you ever chew a lollipop? Though it might seem gratifying in the moment, chomping on hard candy moves the experience along much faster. In effect, we are consuming the same amount of food but with less opportunity to enjoy it than if we were to allow it to dissolve slowly. The more time we give ourselves to enjoy meals, experiences, or activities, the more opportunity we have to enjoy those things. When we focus our attention on what we are doing (or eating), we can be satisfied by the experience with a smaller dose. In other words, less candy, fewer chips, and less soda can satisfy us fully with a much smaller quantity. If you are in a habit of overeating, over-doing screen time, or are out of balance in another area of life, practice savoring the experience.

1 Do you find yourself eating and drinking foods quickly? Once you finish, do you find yourself craving seconds?

2 When you eat your meals today, direct your attention to the pleasurable qualities of what you're eating. Consider the taste, texture, and temperature of the food. Add more salt if the food is bland, or make other adjustments to maximize your enjoyment of your portion. Reflect on how this process increases the satisfaction of your meals in relation to the amount of food you are eating.

Happy: Keep a Gratitude Journal

In the same way that savoring food can increase satisfaction, reflecting on the pleasurable and beautiful aspects of life can increase our enjoyment at work, home, and of life in general. Research shows that spending time expressing gratitude changes the brain on a chemical level, strengthening the neurologic pathways that lead to happiness. The more time we spend intentionally expressing gratitude, the more likely it will be that we will *feel* grateful in the future.

1 Name three things for which you're grateful *right now*. Keep a pad of paper by your bed so that each morning before you sleep you can write down three more, and each night before sleeping you can thank God for his many blessings.

2 What if the only things you had this morning were the things you thanked God for yesterday?

Whole: Read Proverbs Chapter 14

Envy is the antithesis of gratitude. While gratitude is an expression of thankfulness for what we do have, envy curses others for what we don't have. Compared to other classic sins, envy is one that really doesn't make sense in that it cannot actually gratify the beholder. Lies may get us out of trouble, *at least temporarily*. Lust may make us feel good, *at least temporarily*. Wealth may excite us, *at least temporarily*. But coveting the possessions of our neighbors doesn't grant us ownership over those objects. Resenting God for what he has given to our friends doesn't prompt him to bless us likewise. We read in Proverbs 14:30 that "A heart at peace gives life to the body, but envy rots the bones." This statement rings true time and time again. Envy cannot and will not lead to good. But gratitude and grace beget peace, and a peaceful, joyful heart is one that worships God.

1 Do you find that some of your attitudes, behaviors or choices are a reaction to something someone else has that you likewise desire?

2 Sometimes our envious attitudes stem from insecurity, grief, or anger. Consider the things you *covet*. What do you think is behind those desires?

DAY 15

Healthy: Stretch

Movement is life. When we are stagnant, when we fail to grow and move, we inch closer and closer to an empty, still life. Everything we do, every day, requires movement. Our muscles contract, our limbs reach, our feet walk us through life. Muscles that aren't used often become stiff and sore. If exercise is uncomfortable, if you have a crook in your neck, if you're not able to bend forward like you used to, improve your ability to move through life by stretching out your muscles. Stretching is an extremely beneficial but often overlooked health practice. Not only does it help prevent athletic injury, but it can improve energy levels, boost our moods, and even boost our metabolisms. With a minimal time investment (less than five minutes per day) the payoff can be huge: more eagerness and energy to get up, get going, and engage with life!

1 When will you fit in a stretch today? Before exercise? Upon waking? During your break at work?

2 Before stretching, rate your energy level on a scale of 1-10. Spend a minute stretching each arm, each leg, and the muscles around your neck and back. Take a few deep breaths and rate your energy level again. How has it changed?

Happy: Take the Middle Road

Don't start anything today that you can't keep up for the rest of your life. Do you think that you would become happier if you quit your job and moved to a tropical island? How about wellness – would you be healthier if you became a vegan? Maybe, maybe not. But if you're like most people, embarking on such a dramatic lifestyle change would prove unsustainable. Not that you couldn't make it work – anything is possible – but statistically speaking, most of such efforts fizzle out in a few weeks or months. Instead of taking a black-and-white approach to life – stressful work or *no* work, a fast food diet or complete veganism – look to make little changes that are sustainable, which will help you stay in the in-between "gray" area. Eating only cookies isn't healthy, but neither is eating only kale.

1 Do you find yourself gravitating toward extremes? Why do you think that is?

2 Think about a challenge in your life you're looking to tackle. What's the next right step you can take in the next 15 minutes to help you along this journey?

Whole: Read Proverbs Chapter 15

"A gentle answer turns away wrath, but a harsh word stirs up anger." – Proverbs 15:1

When someone has wronged us, nothing seems to feel better in the moment than dropping a snarky retort or cultivating the perfect passive-aggressive response. But hours later, after the argument has quieted, the pain of the hurtful comments settles in and the folly of what felt good in the moment becomes more readily apparent. Indulging someone else's anger – especially if it is unrighteous anger – never ends well. We all become angry at times, but the ways we process that anger (or respond to anger in others) can completely change the outcome of the situation.

When a toddler throws a tantrum and the parents starts yelling, the household dissolves into chaos. When an insult is retaliated, war breaks out. But when a mother lowers her voice and refuses to let loose, control is kept in the home even if the child doesn't immediately quiet down. When an insult is ignored, the accuser loses his ammunition and the battle reaches stagnation. Regardless of the fact that choosing gentleness in a moment of fury doesn't feel as good as letting loose, feeding the fire will destroy the forest.

1 Do you find yourself tempted to lose control in trying situations? Consider the last argument you engaged and consider how it might have transpired differently if a gentle answer on your end was given.

2 Which types of situations tend to push your buttons the most? Spend some time curating gentle and calm responses to your most common triggers so that you are prepared the next time you are tested.

DAY 16

Healthy: Get More Sleep

Our lives are busy, and with lengthy to-do lists, work schedules and family demands, it can be difficult to get enough rest. However, when our sleep suffers, so do the other areas of our lives. Sleeping enough is crucial for lasting health and well-being. *Not* sleeping enough can create increased risk of physical and emotional health problems including weight gain, anxiety, infertility, high blood pressure, and even increased likelihood of developing diabetes.

Not getting enough sleep also increases the body's stress response. In periods of sleep deprivation, the body secretes higher than normal levels of cortisol, which is the body's stress hormone. When cortisol is released into the blood stream, it travels to every part of the body. Long term patterns of high cortisol-release can lead to the health problems described above.

1 One of the most important steps a person can take toward health promotion is getting enough sleep, at the right time of day. Research shows that 8 hours of sleep sometime between the hours of 10 pm and 8 am is optimal for cortisol balance.

2 If you're not getting enough sleep, what is getting in your way? Reflect on the reverse-scheduling activity to see what's taking up your time.

3 How would your life benefit (work, relationships, energy, etc.) if you were better rested? Use this as motivation to make the necessary change in your sleep hygiene.

Happy: Develop a New Bedtime Routine

One of the reasons some folks struggle to sleep enough is because they find themselves unable to *fall* asleep. Sometimes, the reason for this insomnia can be related to their bedtime routine. Looking at a glowing screen or TV at night can interrupt the body's perception of when daytime is and when nighttime is. As much as possible, limit screen time for the hour leading up to your target bedtime. Try to also limit high-energy activities like exercise before bed to foster a calm environment. Instead, be deliberate in seeking out relaxing activities during this time, such as reading a book, spending time with family, drinking a cup of hot tea, or listening to soothing music. A hot bath, deep breathing, stretching, and other hygiene practices are also helpful for relaxation before bedtime.

Try to follow the same pattern every day before bed. With time, starting the bedtime routine will help signal to the brain that the time for rest is coming soon. A bedtime routine can not only help insomniacs fall asleep, but they also report better quality sleep and less stress throughout the day.

1 What's your current bedtime habit? Do you find that these habits are helping promote high-quality sleep, or are they detracting from it?

2 What is one thing you can choose to do tonight before bed that will easily translate into a consistent habit over time?

Whole: Read Proverbs Chapter 16

One of the best blessings we can give to others is a cheerful word that boosts their spirits. Have you ever been around a "Debbie Downer," "Negative Nancy," or "Sarcastic Samuel" for any length of time and found yourself feeling down in the dumps afterwards? Compare that to how you feel after being around someone who is optimistic, encouraging, and keeps a positive attitude even in the midst of trial. Which of these categories of people helps you to feel more joyful and better equipped to handle life's challenges?

Proverbs 16:24 reads, "Gracious words are a honeycomb, sweet to the soul and healing to the bones." When we choose to share words of encouragement with others, we are able to give them a lasting gift that will come to mind for them again and again. Be the reason someone's day is lifted. Choose to put in the effort to share a kind word. A peaceful heart nourishes the soul.

1 When was the last time someone shared an encouragement that completely transformed your day? How can you pay that gift forward *today*?

2 Consider this common saying: "As one person, I can't change the world, but I can change one person's world." Who will you seek to encourage today?

DAY 17

Healthy: Wash Your Face

Even if we don't wear makeup, our faces secrete small amounts of oil throughout the day that easily collect dirt, dust, and bacteria. These can clog pores and lead to pimples, and it can also contribute to a generalized feeling of discomfort. Washing your face can be helpful in waking up for an energized boost to the morning but at the same time, can help foster relaxation in the evening before bed. Face washing is a way to say to yourself, "I care about you!"

By taking care of your skin and dedicating time to self-care, you can cultivate a lasting positive effect on your well-being in less than five minutes. The best part is that it's completely free – just some warm water and a towel. While gentle soap can help clear away oil and grime, there's no need for expensive powders, salves, or creams. The old-fashioned way is truly the best!

When will you wash your face today?

Happy: Rekindle Your Relationships

Life is all about relationships. A life that is lived completely alone is an empty one, as our meaning and purpose is rooted in love and service for God and others. At the same time, in order to thrive in life, we too need relationships that can feed, support, and encourage us! A close social support system is considered one of the primary determinants of well-being. Having two or three individuals who you can rely on in times of need, with whom you can enjoy pastimes, and toward whom you can invest your own time and energy is essential for a healthy social life.

The best way to foster these types of relationships is with regular, intentional time spent together. If you're married or in a relationship, start with your partner. Commit to a weekly date night together, where you tune out the distractions, leave work behind, and invest in each other through honesty and encouraging communication. Date nights don't need to be expensive, either – cook at home, enjoy a leisurely hike together, or play a board game. Anything that gives you face-to-face time will do the job. If you're single, you still need meaningful relationships! (Even married folks need their friends.)

Invest in the lives of those near and dear to you with coffee dates. Spend at least two hours per week investing in important friendships in your life – whether it's a gal pal, your dad, or your siblings, relationships that are neglected fizzle out. If you don't drink coffee, no problem! Share a meal, get together for a "play date" with your kids, work out together, or offer to help with a house project. Whatever it takes, keep up with your friends!

1 Which meaningful relationships in your life have you been neglecting? Who can you call today to catch up, chat, and rekindle your friendship?

2 When can you carve out at least two hours in your week to get together with someone who is important to you? Seek to reach out to at least one person every week.

Whole: Read Proverbs Chapter 17

"A friend loves at all times, and a brother is born for a time of adversity." – Proverbs 17:17

Have you ever heard of the concept of fair-weather friends? Essentially, this refers to people in our lives who are happy to befriend us when everything is going well or if we can improve *their* lives in some way, but who aren't likely to show up when *we* are the ones in need. Suffering in life is unavoidable, but suffering in solitude doesn't have to be.

By coming alongside our loved ones when they are facing struggles, we can be part of the reason they are able to push through. Whether we are meeting a direct need, offering an encouraging word, or simply sitting silently in support, our presence can be life-changing or even life-*saving*.

1 The last time you were facing crisis, who came alongside you to help you through it? These people – the ones who showed up – proved their love and loyalty to you through their support. Have you ever thanked them for their help? Write them a note today.

2 Who in your life is facing hard times right now? How can you show your support to them? What action could you take *today* that would help *you* to be a better friend?

DAY 18

Healthy: Try Something New

Keeping things fresh and interesting keeps us wanting more. Not that there isn't something to be said for structure and routine, but variety is the spice of life. If your exercise habits are too boring to be motivating, it might be time to try something new. Experiment with a novel type of exercise, or a new take on something you know and love. If you typically practice yoga, try hot yoga, aerial yoga, or goat yoga. (Yes, goat yoga is a real thing.)

If yoga isn't your typical choice of exercise, try it out! It might surprise you. At the same time, if you've tried yoga, weightlifting, or water polo and they don't feel so good for you, there's no reason to force yourself to suffer through them. There are countless options for fun, engaging, and feel-good exercise that can empower and energize your life. Likewise, if your exercise habits feel like a terrible chore, experimenting with new experiences may enlighten you to better ways to care for yourself through movement.

1 Do your exercise habits empower you to live life to the fullest? If not, what is one change you can make today to make exercise more enjoyable or convenient?

2 Are you willing to branch out with your exercise and try something new? Why or why not? If not, what's holding you back?

Happy: Try Something New

If not exercise, new hobbies can help keep life fun and interesting. Spruce up your mealtimes by taking a cooking class for a fun way to learn new recipes. Invite a friend for a day trip to a new city and take a bike tour. Sign up for a class about a topic you know nothing about and share what you learned with your family. Take up knitting! Whatever it is, don't settle for stagnation.

Learning new skills is not only enjoyable, but doing so can also empower us to serve others in new ways. We're never too young or too old, too busy or "too much" of anything else to prevent us from diversifying our skillsets. Whether you are learning a new language, becoming CPR certified, or sharing your faith for the first time, be constantly looking for ways to grow yourself.

1 Are you an adventure-seeker or a creature of habit? How long has this been true of you? If you have a more eager spirit, why do you think you are that way?

2 If you prefer routine and predictability, why do you think that is? For you personally, what would be the benefit in learning something new? How would this affect the other people in your life?

3 If everything stayed exactly the same as today for the rest of your life, how would your ability to serve God or others be limited? What can you do today to take steps toward growth?

Whole: Read Proverbs Chapter 18

Nobody likes a know-it-all because, at the end of the day, *nobody* actually knows it all. Even scientific understanding is limited in knowledge. Commonly accepted theories are disproved every day. With the rising and setting of the sun, lies are uncovered, ideas are changed, opinions are swayed. The difference between the foolish and the wise is that the latter group acknowledges the limits of their understanding whereas those in the former deny that they exist. Usually, the reason we share our opinions (at least in unsolicited situations) is because we think we are right, and having superior knowledge makes us feel good. But frankly, dumping our opinions on others rarely is effective at changing *theirs*. In fact, it often does a disservice. All throughout Chapter 18 of Proverbs we read about how the mouths of fools are their undoing. Talking too much gets us into trouble, harming relationships among friends (verses 1 and 8), drowning out opportunity for truth (verse 4) and catching them in contradictions (verse 7). Proverbs 18:2 reads, "Fools find no pleasure in understanding but delight in airing their own opinions." Rather than seeking to show your thoughts to others, cultivate a desire to learn from others.

1 Do you tend to discount others' views, or are you receptive to new ideas? Remember that God is the only one with infinite wisdom. Ask him for guidance and grace in cultivating a humble attitude.

2 The best way to find out what we don't know is to seek out new information. Cultivate curiosity about a new topic and use the excitement and mystery of the unknown to remember that the world is filled with information yet to be dis-

covered.

DAY 19

Healthy: Take a Deep Breath

Say this out loud: "Ommmmmmmmmmmmmm."

What does it make you think of? Monks? Meditation? Deep breathing? Research continues to prove the importance of deep, diaphragmatic breathing – and not just during periods of stress. Proper breathing technique allows our lungs to be filled completely, whereas holding in our tummies and elevating our chests to breathe prevents us from getting full oxygenation. The mechanical action of breathing also stimulates the *rest and digest*, stress-relieving division of our nervous systems, lowering cortisol and changing our health in measurable ways.

Practice Healthy Breathing: To find your breath, lay on your back with your knees bent. Place one hand on your belly and one hand on your chest. When you take a breath, strive to distend your belly so that your hand elevates straight up without moving your ribs to elevate the hand on your chest. You also could practice while you're sitting by cinching your hands around your waist. When you take a breath, strive to increase your abdominal pressure enough to push your hands outward and away from your belly button. Do this as often as you remember, until it becomes "normal" for you.

Happy: Reconcile with Your True Feelings

The vast majority of relationship problems result from poor communication in some way, shape, or form. Whether a person's needs were not being met, there was a misunderstanding, a big decision needed to be made, or whatever the reason – concerns that don't get communicated can't be resolved. However, the necessary precursor to healthy and respectful communication is humble self-awareness.

If we aren't aware of how we are feeling ourselves, we can't hope to communicate that to the other people in our lives. If we don't reconcile ourselves with our true feelings and instead try to stuff them down, ignore them, numb them away, or turn to unhealthy coping mechanisms, we might feel pacified for the moment, but the problem will be left to fester.

1 Which of your own relationship problems have resulted from poor communication? How could have (or did) self-awareness empower you to reconcile with the other people involved in the situation?

2 Consider the issues that afflict you most often in life. Why do these issues affect you as they do? What is going on in your own heart that leads you to perceive the situation as you do? How will you communicate this to others?

Whole: Read Proverbs Chapter 19

"A person's own folly leads to their ruin, yet their heart rages against the Lord." – Proverbs 19:3

When we sign up for a credit card, we are required to submit our social security number. This is because the charges we file on that card will be our own responsibility to pay. If the things we buy with that card are to belong to us, the bill also needs to belong to us. Taking ownership of our possessions requires that we put forth the time, money, or effort to acquire and keep them. The same responsibility falls upon each of us to accept the price of our actions. Whether intentionally or not, everything we do has consequences, whether good or bad. When we are strong and courageous or accomplish something great, the honor and reward is our own. But when we neglect our responsibilities, accrue debt, or miss out on opportunities due to lack of preparation, again the consequences are our own.

This verse from Proverbs pays homage to situations in which a person winds up facing unpleasant consequences as a result of their own actions (or lack thereof). Yet, instead of recognizing their own fault and responsibility, they blame God. Sure, sometimes bad things happen to us and sometimes good things happen to us, and sometimes those things are out of our control. But sometimes, we bring them upon ourselves. If we are unhappy with the result and prefer alternate outcomes in the future, we must accept the responsibility and making changes in ourselves if we are to have any hope of a different tomorrow.

1 Consider your present circumstances – both good and bad. Which of your experiences are the consequences of your own previous actions and attitudes?

2 What can you do today to continue these positive experiences? What can you do today to prevent negative experiences tomorrow?

DAY 20

Healthy: Question Your Cravings

"Am I hungry, or am I bored?" Have you ever found yourself asking this question? Part of honoring our bodies means responding appropriately to our cravings rather than ignoring them. If we try to appease a brownie craving with a chocolate protein shake, for example, the craving might not be satisfied. After eating twelve different "healthy" snacks in an attempt to avoid the brownie, we end up eating far too much and often succumbing to the brownie anyway. By eating a brownie the first time, we can satisfy ourselves and move on with life. But sometimes, the real driver behind the inclination to eat a brownie isn't a craving for chocolate but rather a craving for excitement. In other words, sometimes we are just bored.

Question Your Cravings: If you struggle to identify when you're hungry versus when you're just bored, start with this exercise:

Consider the food you are thinking of eating. Ask yourself how you would feel if you ate this item. Would you feel more energized? Relieved? Pleasantly satiated? Or would you feel too full, lethargic, or overly sugared/salted? Compare this feeling to how you feel when you are hungry and finally eat, or when you're too full but keep eating. Which of these two circumstances seems to be the more likely result?

If you aren't able to identify how you feel in the moment, set a timer for 20 minutes and engage in another activity. Take a shower, a walk, or drink a glass of water. If after 20 minutes you still aren't sure, take a bite and re-evaluate. If it isn't as enjoyable as you imagined, set it aside for later. Food tastes best when it's what we really need in the moment.

Happy: Let Go

Maybe the best next step to cultivate joy in your life isn't adding something new, but rather taking something away. Overflowing junk drawers, clogged closets and cluttered homes can stress us out. Disrespectful or demanding people can weigh heavily on our hearts. Negative ideas, cynical attitudes and pessimistic perspectives can fog our experience of life. Instead of looking for a new purchase or a new relationship, start with your perception.

De-clutter your life by letting go of what you don't need so that you can embrace more of what truly adds value to your life. Whether that means physically throwing items away, setting and maintaining boundaries, or choosing to reject harmful thought patterns, sometimes the key to a happier, healthier life is choosing to live with less.

1 Which physical items are weighing you down? Would you be willing to discard them for a life with less stress?

2 Which relationships in your life could benefit from better reinforcement of boundaries? What would it look like to protect you and your values?

3 Do you have a tendency to succumb to negative or otherwise pessimistic thought patterns? How can you practice interrupting those patterns and cultivate new ones?

Whole: Read Proverbs Chapter 20

"Who can say, 'I have kept my heart pure; I am clean and without sin'?" Proverbs 20:9

Each of us has room to grow. Even if we have been successful in healing in one area of life, there is another habit, attitude, or belief that could use some attention. As much as we might like to think otherwise, we aren't perfect, and realizing those character deficits is only a matter of time. When we view the world around us, we may be tempted to adopt a critical or even judgmental attitude towards other people, condemning them for how they live, what they value, or what they believe. But when we point the finger, we forget that we too are imperfect.

In Matthew 7:3, Jesus says, "Why do you look at the speck of sawdust in your brother's eye and pay no attention to the plank in your own eye?" In other words, he is reminding us that we have no business picking, prodding, and pointing out the imperfections in others because we too have flaws, many of which are screaming for attention.

1 Before condemning others for their shortcomings, spend time reflecting on your own life: in which areas could you stand to grow? Are you guilty of the same sins you notice in others?

2 If you find yourself tempted to believe that you don't have anything pressing to work on, humbly ask God to point out the areas you need to grow. Keep in mind that the answer to this prayer may be an increase in situations that draw out your imperfections. For example: if we are lacking in patience, God may present us with trying situations that give us opportunity to exhibit patience...and so on and so forth.

DAY 21

Healthy: Back to the Basics

If alternative coffee creamer made from almond milk (etc.) is your preference – that's awesome! We all deserve to enjoy our favorite foods. However, if you are choosing these products in the name of health, you might be surprised to learn that they aren't necessarily the healthier choice. Dairy products in particular are under fire in the media and while its true that inflammation related to dairy protein intolerance can exacerbate health problems, milk from a cow is the more natural, less processed option when it comes to coffee additions.

Nut-based coffee creamers have undergone extensive extraction and emulsification processes to achieve the consistency and stability that they have. In making these products, oils are forced into watery solutions, and chemically altered to keep them there. They also usually contain added sugar and artificial flavors to make them more palatable. So, even though almond oil is healthy, almond based "creams" and nut milks aren't necessarily healthy at all.

Half-and-half is actually a more natural and arguably more healthful option for the average, healthy individual, and the same can be said of other types of food products. Fat-free products contain extra sugar, gluten-free baked goods are often far higher in calories and additives, and sugar-free sweets certainly aren't superior to their regular counterparts.

1 Are you choosing alternative health products (without medical necessity like allergies) because you think they are "better" or because you truly enjoy them more? Considering the truth about the relationship between processed food and health, will you continue to choose them?

2 When God created the world, he designed food for human consumption in an intentional way. He didn't make a mistake when he put gluten in bread or sugar in fruit. From this perspective, what do you think God's views are about ultra-processed food products? How should this influence your decisions going forward?

Happy: Be More timely

Traffic is bumper-to-bumper for miles, drivers are shouting, horns are blaring, stress is high. Worst of all, the clock is ticking...time crunches create stress. Waiting until the last minute – even if everything ultimately ends up being on time – creates unnecessary anxiety, fear, or other emotional fallout. A little extra planning and preparation is worth every minute for the margin it creates. When you finally walk into the workplace, is it at the very minute your shift starts? Do you replenish your coffee beans only after you've already run out? Do you wait until after the deadline to file your taxes, become frustrated by the late fees, and groan when your return is less than you'd prefer?

Our responsibilities need to get taken care of, and we always need to end up *doing the thing*...whether we're timely about it or not. So, why not leave a few minutes early each day, put coffee beans on the grocery list when the bag is only half empty, and set a reminder for important deadlines the week *before* they're due? A little extra work on the front end can save us a lot of stress and frustration later on. If you need a new mantra for your agenda, try this one: "Early is on time, on time is late, and late is way too stressful."

1 Are you a timely person? Why or why not? What can you do today to facilitate a lifestyle schedule that contains enough margin to respect your time?

2 What's the next item on your agenda today? Commit right now to starting 5 minutes early.

Whole: Read Proverbs Chapter 21

"It's better to ask for forgiveness than permission."

Have you ever heard that phrase? As tempting as it is to evade authority and sneak under the radar, doing so isn't the best course of action. While it may seem *easier* in the moment, it isn't the *best* course of action. God's word encourages us otherwise in Proverbs 21:3 –

"To do what is right and just is more acceptable to the Lord than sacrifice."

Doing things the right way, the first time, honors God. Even though his grace and mercy are enough to forgive even the greatest of transgressions, following God's instruction and obeying his commands – including that which calls us to submit to authority – is better than asking for forgiveness later. It all comes down to the attitude of our *hearts*.

When we seek to honor God and pursue his will, we are intentional about prayerfully and humbly choosing what we believe God would have us do in the first place. On the contrary, doing what we want and half-heartedly asking forgiveness later demonstrates an attitude of rebellion: we don't *really* want to honor God, we want to honor ourselves! But we likewise want to give the appearance of holiness, so we mutter an "I'm sorry" under our breath, and then carry on our way.

1 When you make decisions, is your first step to consult God or to consult your own desires?

2 Consider the last major decision you made. How could your process have looked differently if your primary concern was holiness rather than self-gratification?

DAY 22

Healthy: Get Up for a Reset

Research shows that prolonged sitting can increase risk of cardiovascular disease, diabetes, and other conditions. But for those of us with desk jobs, activity throughout the day isn't always an option. However, taking breaks after sitting for long periods can be helpful in promoting health by temporarily boosting the heart rate, stretching stiff muscles, and keeping joints loose and mobile.

Any time you find yourself sitting for a long period of time – such as at work or during a long meeting – use break opportunities to stand up, stretch out, and take a lap. Start by stretching out your neck, then your arms, then your back, then your legs. Take a few deep breaths, and then walk back and forth through the longest hallway in the building. If it's nice out, take a lap around the block. If you work in a large building, take a few flights of stairs up and down. After the walk, repeat your quick stretch, and get back to work feeling energized and refreshed!

1 When can you fit in a ten-minute reset today? Where will you do your walk?

2 Commit to taking three breaks from sitting today. Write down what time you will get up, set an alarm or a reminder, write yourself a note – whatever it takes. *Just do it.*

Happy: A Dollar A Day

One of the most common causes of conflict among couples is money. One of the biggest *personal* stressors is finances. One of the greatest contributors to bankruptcy is debt. Financial margin is a big deal. If an apple a day keeps the doctor away, a dollar a day can keep debt away. The average American has $16,000 of credit card debt, nearly $40,000 of student loan debt, and upwards of $245,000 in mortgage borrowing. *Oof*.

With a number that far in the red, it may seem nearly impossible to find enough financial margin to start making *extra* monthly payments. But it is possible. With a dollar a day. By saving one dollar a day towards paying off debt, we can slowly chip away at the monetary mountain. Of course, at this rate, it would take three years to pay off just $1,000. But in the beginning, the amount isn't the biggest factor – it's the principle. (Or perhaps, the principal...)

Starting small starts flexing our saving muscles. It gets us used to doing something other than living paycheck-to-paycheck. It helps us practice setting something aside for later. When we slowly start cutting back on expenses, one dollar easily becomes one dollar more, and another, and another, until paying off debt becomes a reality and building up a savings becomes the norm.

1 To what degree do finances affect your life? Your relationships? Your stress?

2 What can you cut back on *today* to start saving just $1 towards paying off debt or building up savings?

Whole: Read Proverbs Chapter 22

One of the most important applications for wisdom in today's day and age is to the subject of finances. In the modern era, wealth abounds but proper money management is often severely lacking. Current estimates are that nearly 87% of families are in debt with nearly 50% carrying credit card debt. While borrowing money isn't outright prohibited in scripture, the absence of debt is encouraged, and God warns us about the many dangers of debt.

Proverbs 22:7 is a key example of such verses: "The rich rule over the poor and the borrower is slave to the lender." Having debt not only can cause stress, but it can limit our ability to give to others. When we incur more expenses that we can sustain for ourselves, further spending (even for charity) is inherently unwise. Debt limits us from generosity. Debt also limits work options: we must seek employment that compensates us enough for living expenses as well as for debt repayment. We cannot move to new places, seek new experiences, or enjoy the same degree of flexibility and freedom as those without debt if we personally are enslaved to lenders.

1 Have you ever owed someone something? How did it make you feel to be in that position?

2 Are you currently in debt? How does this affect your relationship with God? How can you approach your debt in a way that honors God?

3 What would the benefit of debt-free living be for you, in your current situation?

DAY 23

Healthy: Make Freezer Meals

Eating healthy has a bad reputation: expensive, time consuming, challenging, inconvenient, *boring*. Have you ever thought those things yourself, then headed out to a restaurant or fast food joint for something easy, quick, and cheap? But what if, when you walked through the door of your home, you could take off your shoes, unpack your bag, shower, and then settle down just in time for a delicious, hot meal, fresh out of the oven? With just a few minutes of preparation and intention, you can.

Next time you are preparing a recipe – whether it's a casserole for church, lasagna for Sunday dinner, or some old fashioned, slow-cooked pot roast – double the recipe. But instead of overloading your fridge with leftovers, freeze them. Before cooking the second lasagna, wrap the pan in plastic wrap and freeze it. Before throwing the second batch of slow-cooker ingredients into the pot, put them in a freezer bag...and then the freezer. First thing when you come home from work (or first thing in the morning if it's for the slow-cooker) unwrap the casserole, put it in the oven at the usual temperature, and cook for an additional 30 minutes, or until the inside is hot and cooked through. By the time you're all set and ready to eat, your dinner will be, too.

1 How often do you find yourself stopping at fast food restaurants out of convenience? Make it your goal to cut that number down by 50% this month.

2 What is the next meal you plan to cook at home? Commit to doubling the ingredients and putting an extra portion in the freezer.

3 If you're more of a recipe follower than an intuitive cook, that's okay! There are thousands of recipes of freezer-to-oven ready recipes online with easy steps, beautiful pictures, and delicious flavor. Browse around and find something you like!

Happy: Create More Margin

"Busy and tired." Is that how you answer when someone asks you how you're doing? Really, that's how most of us answer. In fact, that's generally the *expected* answer. Most folks today are overscheduled and overworked, tired, frazzled, and with little margin in their lives. Margin is unscheduled time. Margin is breathing room. Margin is freedom.

Too little time in our schedules can make us slaves to them. Instead of being the ones in charge of our lives, we are overcome by our commitments in life. We become like robots instead of truly living. There are two ways to cultivate margin in life: set the boundaries around margin (a pre-scheduled time) and allow commitments to fall outside of that; or, set boundaries around responsibilities and use the remaining available time for margin.

1 When you are asked to make commitments, do you have a hard time saying no? Are these commitments infringing on the margin in your life?

2 Are the responsibilities in your life so demanding that free time isn't an option?

3 Which of these responsibilities can you cut back on, eliminate, or streamline to free up margin in your life?

4 What do you think are the consequences of a margin-less life?

Whole: Read Proverbs Chapter 23

"Do not wear yourself out to get rich; do not trust your own cleverness." – Proverbs 23:4

In the book of Proverbs, we often read of warnings against laziness, neglect, and lack of diligence. While indulging these qualities can certainly set us up for disaster, there is risk of swinging to the opposite end of the spectrum, too. We can turn work into an idol, worshipping wealth and obsessing over the bottom line. In the blink of an eye, all our worldly wealth can disappear. Our cars can be totaled. Our homes can be burned down. We could lose our jobs. If all our time investments are been centered around acquiring wealth with little margin for anything else, we are living an empty life. God is not *against* wealth, work, or hard work. However, his desire for us is to cultivate lives of freedom, where we aren't enslaved to the *pursuit* of wealth, aren't captivated by *love* for wealth, and that don't enslave us to expensive lifestyles that limit our ability to create lives characterized by love and service.

1 Does your life have enough margin in terms of time and finances to allow you to love and serve others with freedom? If not, what is holding you back?

2 What is your mindset when you consider your money? Is your primary goal to earn and save, to purchase things you want and like, to cultivate margin for experiences or generosity, to pay off debt?

3 How does your mindset align (or not) with your faith?

DAY 24

Healthy: Tuck Your Chin

When you think about health and well-being, how often does posture come to mind? Do you typically regard posture as more of an aesthetic consideration or an aspect of physical health? Sure, healthy, straight posture is an appealing physical quality. But there are also health consequences from poor posture that can potentially be debilitating to life. This includes headaches or migraines, increased risk of disc herniations, decreased abdominal core strength and subsequent risk of abdominal hernias, back pain, neck pain, or other physical dysfunctions.

In the age of the opioid epidemic, maintaining good posture and musculoskeletal stability is essential in preventing physical injury, pain syndromes, and the need for prescription drugs with a high risk of addition. Many of life's general aches and pains can be attributed to poor posture. Have you ever woken up with a stiff neck from sleeping in an abnormal position? This is an example of how prolonged abnormal or incorrect posture can create physical problems. When we are awake and sitting, standing, or walking with dysfunctional biomechanics, we are subjecting our bodies to abnormal stresses that they can't withstand for long before pain starts to emerge.

1 When you sit, do you typically slump over, lean to the side, or hunch? Or, are you unsure about the quality of your posture, but you have nonspecific aches and pains after sitting

for long periods of time?

2 To help improve posture, use a top-to-bottom approach by beginning with your neck. Whether you're sitting, standing, walking, driving, or anything else, you can complete this simple exercise to improve your neck posture:

3 Begin by looking straight ahead. Relax your shoulder sand make your neck as straight as possible. (Think about this as trying to reach the top of your head as closely as you can to the ceiling.) Then, using your first two fingers to push the front of your chin straight backwards, essentially tucking your chin towards your chest so that the back of your neck elongates. Repeat this exercise in sets of 10 as often as you think of it.

Happy: Experiences > Stuff

The difference between *stuff* and *experiences* is that *stuff* sticks around long after it's purchased but only brings joy for a short period of time. In other words, the thrill is in the purchase. On the other hand, *experiences* last only a short time, but bring lasting memories that can enrich the experience of life. Think about the Christmas gifts you received this past year. How many of them were physical objects, and how many of those are things you use on a daily basis? This *stuff* gets lost, broken, or out of style. Ultimately, we end up forgetting all about them.

On the other hand, our experiences in life stick with us, shaping us into who we are, offering (hopefully) joyful memories that last forever. Our stuff stays with us for a season, but our life experiences are timeless. Memories of visiting new places, spending time with loved ones, and learning new skills are things that can never be taken away from us. They are treasures of our hearts that will last forever. Experiences are also often social. A friend or family member can join you for a cooking class, accompany you to a zoo, share a delicious meal, or visit breathtaking sights on vacations. But many of the stuff we own is self-centered: our clothes, trinkets, or trendy items.

1 What are some of your favorite memories in life? Are these memories centered around *stuff* or special *experiences*?

2 Do you tend to give (or request) gifts that are material goods or that are life experiences? What would it look like to change this focus towards a gift that keeps on giving?

Whole: Read Proverbs Chapter 24

"Do not gloat when your enemy falls; when they stumble, do not let your heart rejoice." -- Proverbs 24:17

Who do you consider to be your enemy? While real life isn't much like a supervillain story, we all face opposition: fellow athletes in a race, competitors in a job application process, the opposing team. Do you feel a sense of vindication when the high school jock gets dumped? When the annoying colleague gets fired? When the captain of your team's rival breaks his arm and is forced to take medical leave? Do you wish harm upon those who wrong you? These feelings are normal. They are natural. They are expected. But they do not reflect the goodness, kindness, and mercy of God.

The way we view our enemies – even enemies in the silliest of circumstances – is a testament to our own true character. See, behind the rat race, underneath the uniform, below the surface of social status, people are still people, and all people are loved by God. The truth is that sometime people act wrongly. Sometimes they are contrarian, annoying, or inconvenient, just as we are. But when we loathe them, curse them, or wish ill upon them, we are acting in accordance with our evil desires. When we humble ourselves and our own comfort and desires, choosing instead to see even our enemies as beloved children of God, we are then reflecting the higher calling of our faith in Christ.

1 Consider a person in your life who frustrates you. They could be a close personal contact or even someone distant from you. In what light do you typically think of this person?

2 What would it take to change your perspective towards your enemies? What barriers would you need to overcome?

DAY 25

Healthy: Choose Your Joy

If it isn't healthy or delicious, why eat it? By choosing foods that we truly enjoy (or that we know are very important for health, like green vegetables) we can maximize the experience of eating without overloading ourselves. When something is *highly* satisfying, we need less of it to meet our needs. But when something doesn't taste good, we tend to keep eating it in hopes that the next bite might be better than the last. Instead of settling for mediocre choices, be intentional about cooking foods you love. Likewise, for healthy foods that you eat more for functional reasons, take care to season them in a way that isn't just *fine* -- season them to be truly delicious. Then, when you walk away from the meal, you'll be set free to start thinking about something other than the satisfaction you *didn't* get from food.

Ask yourself the following questions to help guide your food choices in terms of what, when, and how much to eat:

1 What is my hunger level right now? If I eat now, will I be hungry enough to share in the next meal or snack? If I don't eat now, will I have the energy I need to sustain me through the rest of my day?

2 What food will taste satisfying right now? Which foods will provide my body with lasting energy until my next meal or snack?

Happy: Clean Up Your Phone

Do you every find yourself with a sore neck after hunching over your phone for an extended period of time? "Tech neck" is an increasingly common complaint among people of all ages. The reason for this is, of course, the fact that we are collectively using our phones *way too much*. This isn't to say that things like email, apps, and other functions are inherently bad. Many of them are useful and make our lives much easier! However, the mode of access (phones) is harming us because of the frequency and duration of time spent looking down.

Another downside to having phones with an enormous number of functional capabilities is *distraction*. The more we look at our phones (even for good reasons) the more opportunity we have to become distracted. Texts capture our attention, emails buzz through the day, and advertisements pop up all over the screen. These things can stress us out, interrupt our focus and subsequent productivity, and have an overall negative effect on our sense of well-being. A life with *less* technology is often a life that is *more* fulfilling. The best way to combat these sorts of distractions is to use technology in your life differently.

Instead of using your phone for email, reading, or banking, switch as many of these daily functions over to a computer as you can. By deleting apps from your phone, it creates incentive to look *up* at a computer screen, to read a book instead of squint at glowing fine print, or maybe to do something altogether tech-free. Sure, phones are convenient for things like banking, but using a computer forces us to be more intentional about our time spent online. It's also much better for our posture, and paper pages of a book are easier on our eyes than the blue light screens.

Deleting phone apps may seem irritating for the first few days, but as time passes, symptoms of tech neck will subside, eye strain will diminish, and countless hours of distraction will be eliminated.

1 Do you find yourself constantly checking your phone throughout the day? How does this affect your posture? Your productivity? Your well-being?

2 How many apps are currently on your phone? Make a goal to cut that number by 50%. Today.

Whole: Read Proverbs Chapter 25

Have you ever been on a diet or a fast only to give up and overdo it on all the foods of which you'd been depriving yourself? Overindulging the pleasures of life can make us sick. Too much leisure can make us lazy. Too much rich food can breed gluttony. Too much money can give way to the false belief that we have all we need, even without God.

Proverbs 25:16 reads: "If you find honey, eat just enough – too much of it, and you will vomit."

The most obvious application of this verse is as support for self-control and restriction. But an often-neglected understanding of this passage is that it isn't saying that life's pleasures on their own are bad. It's merely paying homage to the risk of indulging *excessively*. Do you find yourself believing that dessert is "bad" and therefore feeling a sense of guilt for indulging in it? Or do you feel ashamed for enjoying your favorite TV show once per week?

Consuming media, sweets, and other treats is part of enjoying life's pleasures. Self-denying pleasure and enjoyment on principle is not endorsed by God. Rather, he invites us to enjoy – "Taste and see," he tells us, "That [I am] good!" (Psalm 34:8). Eating and enjoying *too much* isn't healthful, but neither is asceticism – the practice of abstinence from worldly pleasures.

1 When you indulge in your favorite pleasures, do you feel guilty and ashamed, or do you lean into an attitude of gratitude for them?

2 How could focusing *more* on your enjoyment of God's provision deepen your faith and empower *more* moderate and balanced living?

DAY 26

Healthy: Drink Less Alcohol

Current research estimates that a glass or two of red wine each week can be health-promoting. Red wine contains powerful antioxidants that can boost cardiovascular health, lower inflammation, and even prevent dementia. But most people, when they drink, aren't choosing just a glass or two of red wine. Most folks drink a wide variety of alcoholic beverages, including those containing artificial flavorings, added sugar, and other highly-processed ingredients.

Many times, we don't choose these drinks because we're seeking to enjoy the finer things in life, but rather because we think it's the sociable thing to do. Indeed, sharing a delicious beverage with a close friend or to celebrate a joyous event is part of life. There's nothing wrong with enjoying alcohol. But are you enjoying it too much? Are you consuming more than the recommended <u>upper</u> limit of one drink daily for women and two drinks for men? Are you choosing options that offer you an interesting and uplifting gourmet experience or are you turning to alcohol because you don't know how else to de-stress?

Even though red wine is understood to potentially offer health benefits, drinking wine isn't the only way to receive those same benefits. In fact, the health risks of too much alcohol can far outweigh the benefits. Alcohol is high in calories, dehydrates us, can deplete energy levels, create dependency, and lead to other health problems. Again, alcohol can be part of a balanced lifestyle, but all of us would benefit from cutting back a little -- no matter how moderately we are already drinking.

1 How many alcoholic beverages do you consume each week? Why do you find yourself choosing those beverages when you do?

2 What would be the benefit in your life of decreasing your alcohol consumption?

Happy: Read a Book

Where do you do most of your reading? Online? The newspaper? Apps on your phone? Do you read nothing at all? Reading a book may seem old-fashioned or childish, but there are countless benefits to getting back to the basics and reading regular books, even for modern adults. For one, reading offers mental stimulation. Whereas TV shows and movies are more passive, reading or listening to audiobooks keeps our mental gears turning and can keep us sharp as we age.

Reading is also an excellent healthy way to reduce stress. A good story is pleasurable, focusing on the task of reading helps us forget the stress of the day, and it gives us a new topic of conversation for others in our lives. Another benefit of reading books is that it allows us to keep learning. Reading allows for vocabulary expansion, better writing skills, and allows us to learn about new subjects. (This is even true with fiction and novels!) Reading has other cognitive benefits, too: improved analytical skills, improved focus and concentration, and increased short term and long term memory are just a few examples.

1 Did you enjoy reading as a child? Do you still regularly read books now? If not, why do you think that is?

2 What would you need to do to start rekindling a reading practice? Which book will you read? When will you read it? What other daily practice might you need to cut back on to incorporate reading?

Whole: Read Proverbs Chapter 26

Do you ever find yourself falling into the same bad habit, or suffering the consequences of repeating the 1same types of offense? Perhaps you have a habit of speeding and have accrued hundreds of dollars in fines for speeding tickets. Maybe you have been involved in more than one fender-bender due to texting and driving or other distractions. Maybe you are single, and find yourself gravitating towards the same sort of abusive or unkind partners who end up hurting you in the same way every time. Or perhaps you find yourself hurting the feelings of your spouse, child, or sibling in the same way -- time and time again. One of the most obvious marks of a lack of wisdom is the tendency of someone to repeat their same mistakes. As Proverbs 26:11 reads, "As a dog returns to its vomit, so fools repeat their folly." In other words, it's a sign of foolishness to make a mistake, reap the negative consequences, and then repeat the same offense.

1 Do you tend to get yourself into trouble for the same things over and over again?

2 Why do you think that is? What do you need to do differently?

DAY 27

Healthy: Honor Your Feelings
Without Using Food

Have you ever tried to unscrew something with a paper clip or bobby pin because you needed a screwdriver but didn't have one? The clip or pin might have gotten the job done, but not as effectively as the original tool would have been able to. Emotional eating is the same way. The truth of the matter is that eating sweets or snacks to soothe uncomfortable emotions feels good. We truly do feel better afterwards, but only for a short while. Within a few hours or days, it becomes readily apparent that food didn't fix the problem. It was just a band-aid, covering the wound without healing it.

Taking care of ourselves means accurately identifying what we need and then responding appropriately to those needs. For those of us who bottle up feelings and emotions, identifying our needs for social relationships, entertainment, friendship, or a good cry might not come easily. However, practice makes progress!

1 When you feel yourself wrestling with uncomfortable feelings, pause for a moment and try to put a name to the emotion. If you struggle with this, writing a few reflective sentences may help, or calling a trusted friend to verbally process for a few minutes.

2 Once you've identified what you're feeling, seek to respond appropriately. If you're lonely, call someone. If you're sad, try journaling. If you're angry, acknowledge the problem and take steps toward resolving the problem. And, of course, if you're truly hungry, eat!

Happy: Screen-Free Sunday

Cutting back on screen time isn't always easy. Many of us find ourselves wrestling with a sort of nervous twitch – the desire to distract ourselves, kill time, or get an entertainment boost. In these moments, putting away our phones can feel agonizing. Practice building your screen-free skills by taking a sabbath from technology once per week. Sundays tend to work best, as we have fewer computer-related demands (such as work) that require our time and attention, and we typically have friends and family more readily available to help us fill the technology-free space.

1 When you're in line at the grocery store, enduring a restaurant wait list, or stuck in traffic, do you find yourself wrestling with technology twitch? Have you always felt this way during waiting periods? If not, why do you think that changed?

2 Make a list of 10 things you can do this weekend instead of watching TV, internet surfing, or scrolling social media on your phone.

Whole: Read Proverbs Chapter 27

When we are sad or lonely, brownies aren't going to solve the problem. When we're suffering from technology twitch, picking up our phones isn't going to make the twitch go away – especially because the true cause of our discomfort is most certainly not technology *deprivation.* In Proverbs 27:7 we read, "One who is full loathes honey from the comb, but to the hungry even what is bitter tastes sweet." When we are able to use food, technology, leisure, and other pleasures as they were intended to be used, they satisfy us. But when we try to substitute them for other needs such as spiritual satisfaction, we end up frustrated and unfulfilled. Eating honey when our stomachs are already full doesn't end well, and neither does adding more technology to a technology twitch. "But to the hungry, even what is bitter tastes sweet."

1 Where in your life are you tempted to use these sorts of misappropriated coping skills?

2 How can you better respond to needs in your life in a way that is more effective and more honoring to who God made you?

DAY 28

Healthy: Go Fish!

Have you ever heard of the concept of healthy fats? As humans, we need to include oils in our diets to maintain good health. Our hearts use fat for fuel, our hormones are made completely from fat, and many essential vitamins and minerals are only found in fatty foods. However, for optimal well-being, simply eating *enough* fat isn't the whole picture; we also need to include fats in the right balance. The area that most of us are lacking is in terms of our omega-3 intake.

Omega-3 fatty acids are unsaturated fats, making them liquid at room temperature. (Consider this in contrast to butter and coconut oil, which are solid at room temperature.) Fatty acids are long chains of carbon atoms linked together with molecular bonds to hydrogen. Unsaturated fatty acids are different from saturated fatty acids because they have fewer hydrogen atoms attached to the chain, and we use names like "omega-6" or "omega-3" to identify which hydrogen atom is "missing."

However, the structure of an omega-3 fatty acid is less important than its *function* in the human body. When we don't get enough of these fatty acids in our diets, our health suffers. But restoring the balance of omega-3's can prevent many of the debilitating diseases that are plaguing our nation today. The best sources of omega-3 fatty acids are fish, chia seeds, hemp seeds, and walnuts. The current recommendations encourage adults to consume at least two servings of fish each week.

1 Do you consume fish regularly? If not, have you heard about the importance of eating fish before? If you have, why do you think fish isn't a part of your routine?

2 If you don't enjoy eating fish, try experimenting with a new recipe. If you don't like it baked, try fried, grilled, or in a salad. If you absolutely cannot stomach it, consider talking to your doctor about taking a fish oil supplement.

Happy: Organize Something

Digging through a junk drawer for a single headache can be an exasperating experience – especially when you can't find it. So, you move on to the next disorganized drawer, then the next, then the next, until you suddenly realize it might be in the closet... When everything has its own home, we know exactly where to look and find what we need the first time – every time. Organization efforts truly can start small. Whether it's a single drawer, a large closet, or the entire kitchen, take it one step at a time. Here's a fool-proof method for tidying up that is systematic and effective:

1) Take everything out of the drawer, closet, or container.
2) Sort through the items as essentials versus non-essentials. Throw away as many non-essentials as you can bear to part with.
3) Group the remaining items according to function and size. Put small items into containers so they remain grouped.
4) Place everything back into the drawer, closet, or container.

1 Do you find your home to be cluttered and chaotic? What do you think is the driving factor behind this? Too much stuff? Too little time?

2 Commit to starting with one: which area of your life will you organize today?

Whole: Read Proverbs Chapter 28

Proverbs 28:18 reads: "The one whose walk is blameless is kept safe, but the one whose ways are perverse will fall into the pit." Reading this, some of us may tempted to find the false hope that as Christians, we are immune to suffering. But the truth is that we are subject to hardship, challenges, persecution and disaster just like anybody else. What this verse is referring to is not those happenings in life that are outside of our control but rather those which are – things like physical well-being, righteous and holy living, acting kindly and patiently in our relationships, and maintaining conservative spending habits to prevent debt.

There are certain things in life – actions, habits, and attitudes – that almost inevitably lead to disaster, whether the consequences are immediately apparent or not. Things like gossip, greed, laziness and other sins lead to problems in life that were otherwise completely avoidable. Some may respond to these observations by saying, "God helps those who help themselves," but a better way to understand it would be like this: "God provides us with the wisdom we need to make the right choices."

1 What are some of the times in your life when you reaped the appropriately negative consequences of your mistakes?

2 How would you communicate to others the benefit and utility of the wisdom we find in the bible?

DAY 29

Healthy: DIY Standing Desk

Have you ever stopped to consider why we sit down to use a computer? Granted, it is arguably more comfortable, but realistically we could just as easily stand to do our work. If the world was set up to have our desks at arm level when we are standing, we'd have improved posture, boost our metabolisms, and maintain our energy. Another way to combat the health effects of sitting sedentary for eight hours each day is to not sit down at all. Or, rather, sit less.

Various furniture companies have realized the need for standing-height types of desks and computer platforms, and some have even created collapsible, adjustable-height platforms that can be placed on top of a desk and calibrated to the user's height. Some companies even make walking desks, which are essentially limited-pace treadmills that allow slow walking while working at the same time. Walking desks are a fun alternative, but they are cost-prohibitive for many. Even the "standing desk" platforms can be prohibitively expensive – but they don't need to be. You can build your own!

DIY Standing Desk: Small stools can be purchased for less than $10 at hardware and department stores. Once you find a stool that is the right height, you can place it on your desk, and then your laptop right on top! Alternatively, you can purchase a larger platform such as fiberglass or finished, recycled wood to place on top of the stool for a larger work surface. Secure the platform with super glue, screws, or just leave it as-is for easy disassembly.

Happy: Focus Forward

Have you ever been in such a rush that you breezed straight past a dear friend walking towards you, without noticing them? Over-scheduled, high-stress, rushed lifestyles can leave us too frazzled and distracted to see what God has brought into our paths. We may walk right over opportunities or ignore those who are close to us because we left our minds at work, or we are too wrapped up with anxious thoughts about the future. Sometimes the ways that God captures our attention is through loud and obvious means: a job offer, a fast-selling house, a sudden and jarring event; but sometimes his ways are much gentler. In these instances, we need to slow down, stop talking, and listen.

Many times the purpose God has for us is rooted in relationship. There's a hurting soul in front of us who we could encourage, serve, or love. Sometimes they're sitting quietly in a corner, but our noses are buried in work. Sometimes it's the people here and now in our lives, but we are preoccupied with the future or with our fantasies. Sometimes it's the mundane of our current lives, but we are distracted by past regrets.

1 What do you spend most of your day thinking about? Is it the task, people, or responsibilities in front of you, or are you preoccupied with other ideas?

2 What current circumstances do you often ignore due to other distractions? Are any of these tasks, responsibilities, or people deserving of more of your attention?

Whole: Read Proverbs Chapter 29

Do you tend to worry what others think, and seek to make choices that you think will be received well by others, or will earn you high praise? Further, do you ever make choices that compromise your values on account of pressures from other people? Proverbs 29:25 reads, "Fear of man will prove to be a snare, but whoever trusts in the lord is kept safe." When we seek human approval for our actions, we will constantly find ourselves falling short.

We can never live up to the expectations of others because every time we seek to please one group, there will be another waiting to criticize us. Political discussions are a perfect example of this: sharing views that align with one party will be completely torn to pieces by the other party. At the end of the day, making choices simply to earn esteem from others will lead to an empty life -- we will compromise our values, our ability to live authentically, and our ability to live up to the unique callings of God on our lives.

1 Are you a people-pleaser? Why do you think that is?

2 What would it look like to seek God's approval with the same degree of eagerness and persistence?

DAY 30

Healthy: Seventh Inning Stretch

When sitting down to a meal, we can easily find ourselves overeating if, instead of intuitively monitoring our hunger and fullness cues, we zone out, distract ourselves, and mindlessly shovel food into our mouths until the portion is gone. However, expecting to dedicate our full, undivided attention to every forkful is unreasonable -- especially if we are dining with other people. What we can do instead to facilitate this sense of awareness without enslaving ourselves to isolated eating experiences is with a mid-meal break.

Pause and Reflect: Halfway through each meal, pause, set down your fork, and take a few deep breaths. Reflect on the pleasurable aspects of your food, your hunger and fullness levels, and whether you'd like to keep eating. Then, proceed accordingly.

Happy: Spend Time in Nature

The University of Minnesota recently published research regarding the mental health benefits of spending time outside in nature. The scientists report findings of reduced fear, anger and stress, and increased feelings of pleasure and peace. "Exposure to nature not only makes you feel better emotionally," they write, "it contributes to your physical well-being, reducing blood pressure, heart rate, muscle tension, and the production of stress hormones."

Most of our lives are spent inside. We sleep inside, eat inside, work inside (usually), study inside, and many of our preferred hobbies are indoor activities. But the great outdoors has so much to offer in terms of mental and physical health benefits, hobbies, exercise, and new experiences. National parks serve as free entertainment, mountains and beach air refresh the spirit, and leisurely walks outside are a wonderful way to de-stress after a long day. Outdoor activities are also diverse in that they can appeal to extroverts and introverts alike. There truly is something for everyone to enjoy.

1 How much time do you spend outside in a given week? Is this less than or more than you would like?

2 What other types of activities use up time in your day that could otherwise be spent outside enjoying nature?

3 Consider the health benefits of being in nature. Are things like reduced stress, improved emotions, decreased blood pressure and reduced muscle tension things that would benefit your own well-being right now?

4 Commit to spending one hour outside this week. What will you do? Who will you invite to join you? Where will you go?

Whole: Read Proverbs Chapter 30

"Every word of God is flawless; He is a shield to those who take refuge in him." – Proverbs 30:5

Throughout this book, we have discussed different aspects and applications of wisdom as presented in the book of Proverbs. However, as is likely readily apparent from reading the different chapters, thirty individual verses comprise only a minute portion of the vast expanse of wisdom available to us in God's word.

The Lord God -- the creator of the world and author of life -- possesses wisdom that surpasses human understanding. While his words may not always make sense to us, may leave us with questions, or wrestling with conviction, we must always remember that his ways are best, and he knows us more deeply and thoroughly than we could ever dream to know ourselves. In light of this, in spite of our questions and limited understanding, our primary desire as Christians should be to "seek refuge in him" -- to seek him above all else.

The first place we look for wisdom should always be God himself -- whether that means dedicated prayer, earnest searching through scripture, or consulting trusted counselors in the faith whose advice we know is consistent with the calling of Christ on our lives.

1 Do you ever find yourself wrestling with questions or unknowns in your faith? Where do you turn in those times? Do you lean closer to God or do you pull away from him?

2 Consider the times in your life when you have seen God's protection and shield in a tangible way. How does remembering this strengthen your faith?

3 Prior to reading through *Healthy, Happy, Whole*, had you studied the book of Proverbs for yourself? Are there other books of the bible you haven't read?

4 How does knowing the importance of God's wisdom and where you can find it influence your desire to spend time reading the bible?

ABOUT

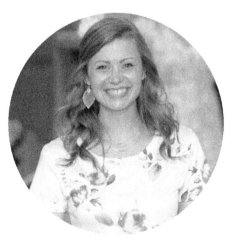

Alexandra MacKillop is a food scientist and primary health-care provider at a holistic clinic near Chicago, IL. She is passionate about helping women cultivate lifestyle behaviors that honor both God and their bodies through a non-diet approach to nutrition and wellness. In addition to clinical practice, she writes about her experiences with faith, food, and medicine on her blog, AlexandraMacKillop.com. Through her writing, she ultimately seeks to encourage others to love God and live fully for Him.

Bible passages in this devotional are from the New International Version (NIV).

Made in the USA
Monee, IL
29 August 2020